BALANITIS

UNDERSTANDING CAUSES, DIAGNOSIS, TREATMENT, AND PREVENTION

DR. J.P JUDE

Table of Contents

CHAPTER ONE

Introduction

Balanitis is a common inflammatory condition that affects the foreskin and head of the penis (glans) in males. It can occur at any age and is characterized by redness, swelling, itching, and pain in the affected area. Balanitis can be acute (short-term) or chronic (long-term) and may result from various causes, including poor hygiene, bacterial or fungal infections, skin conditions, or irritants.

Understanding the symptoms, risk factors, and treatment options for balanitis is essential for proper diagnosis and management of this condition. Prompt medical evaluation and appropriate care can help alleviate symptoms, prevent complications, and promote healing.

In this overview, we'll explore the common causes, symptoms, diagnosis, and treatment options for balanitis, as well as preventive measures to reduce the risk of developing this inflammatory condition. If you or someone you know is experiencing symptoms suggestive of balanitis, it's crucial to consult with a healthcare professional for a comprehensive evaluation and personalized treatment plan.

Definition and Types of Balanitis

Balanitis is an inflammatory condition that affects the foreskin and head of the penis (glans).

It is characterized by redness, swelling, itching, and discomfort in the affected area. Balanitis can be acute, which means it occurs suddenly and lasts for a short period, or chronic, where symptoms persist or recur over an extended period.

Types of Balanitis:

Balanitis

Generalized Balanitis: Inflammation of the foreskin and glans, often associated with poor hygiene, bacterial or fungal infections, or irritants.

Recurrent Balanitis: Chronic or recurrent inflammation of the foreskin and glans due to underlying conditions like phimosis (tight foreskin), diabetes, or dermatological conditions.

Candidal Balanitis (Yeast Infection)

Caused by Candida species (commonly Candida albicans), which are types of yeast that can overgrow in warm and moist environments, leading to infection and inflammation of the foreskin and glans.

Bacterial Balanitis

Bacterial Infection: Caused by bacteria such as Streptococcus or Staphylococcus species, leading to inflammation and infection of the foreskin and glans.

Sexually Transmitted Infections (STIs): Some bacterial STIs, such as syphilis or chlamydia, can cause balanitis.

Contact Dermatitis

Irritant Contact Dermatitis: Inflammation of the foreskin and glans due to exposure to irritants, such as soaps, detergents, condoms, or topical medications.

Allergic Contact Dermatitis: Allergic reaction to substances like latex, spermicides, or personal care products, leading to inflammation and skin irritation.

Zoon's Balanitis (Plasma Cell Balanitis)

A rare type of chronic balanitis characterized by shiny, smooth patches or plaques on the glans, often seen in older uncircumcised men.

Dermatological Conditions

Psoriatic Balanitis: Inflammation and scaling of the foreskin and glans associated with psoriasis.

Lichen Planus: Chronic inflammatory condition causing purple, itchy, flat-topped bumps on the foreskin and glans.

Understanding the specific type of balanitis is essential for proper diagnosis and targeted treatment. A healthcare professional can evaluate the symptoms, perform necessary tests, and determine the underlying cause to develop an appropriate treatment plan tailored to individual needs.

If you or someone you know is experiencing symptoms of balanitis, such as redness, swelling, itching, or discomfort in the genital area, it's crucial to consult with a healthcare professional for an accurate diagnosis and personalized treatment recommendations. Early intervention and appropriate care can help alleviate symptoms, prevent complications, and promote healing.

Common Causes of Balanitis

Balanitis can be caused by a variety of factors, including infections, skin conditions, poor hygiene, irritants, and underlying health conditions. Identifying the underlying cause is crucial for effective treatment and prevention of balanitis. Here are some common causes of balanitis:

1. Poor Hygiene

Inadequate Cleaning: Not cleaning the penis regularly, especially under the foreskin, can lead to the accumulation of smegma (a mixture of oil and dead skin cells) and bacteria, increasing the risk of inflammation and infection.

2. Infections

Bacterial Infections: Bacteria like Streptococcus or Staphylococcus species can cause balanitis, often secondary to poor hygiene or minor injuries.

Yeast Infections (Candidal Balanitis): Overgrowth of Candida species, commonly Candida albicans, in warm and moist environments, such as under the foreskin, leading to infection and inflammation.

3. Skin Conditions

Dermatitis: Contact dermatitis or allergic dermatitis due to exposure to irritants (e.g., soaps, detergents, condoms, topical medications) or allergens (e.g., latex, spermicides, personal care products).

Psoriasis: Chronic skin condition characterized by red, scaly patches that can affect the genital area.

Lichen Planus: Inflammatory skin condition causing purple, itchy, flat-topped bumps on the skin, including the penis and foreskin.

4. Irritants

Chemical Irritants: Exposure to irritants like soaps, perfumes, dyes, or topical medications can cause irritation, inflammation, and allergic reactions.

Physical Irritants: Friction from tight clothing, condoms, or vigorous sexual activity can lead to irritation and inflammation of the foreskin and glans.

5. Underlying Health Conditions

Diabetes: Poorly controlled diabetes can increase the risk of balanitis due to elevated glucose levels promoting bacterial or fungal growth and impaired immune response.

Phimosis: Tight foreskin that cannot be retracted can lead to poor hygiene, accumulation of smegma, and increased risk of inflammation and infection.

Sexually Transmitted Infections (STIs): Some STIs, such as herpes, syphilis, or chlamydia, can cause balanitis.

6. Other Factors

Age: Older men, especially those who are uncircumcised, may be at higher risk due to reduced immune response, decreased elasticity of the foreskin, and increased susceptibility to skin conditions.

CHAPTER TWO

Medications: Some medications, such as antibiotics, antifungal agents, or corticosteroids, can disrupt the natural balance of microorganisms on the skin and mucous membranes, leading to inflammation or infection.

Understanding the common causes of balanitis is essential for prevention, early diagnosis, and targeted treatment. Maintaining good hygiene, avoiding irritants, practicing safe sex, managing underlying health conditions, and seeking prompt medical attention for symptoms can help reduce the risk of developing balanitis and promote genital health and well-being. If you or someone you know is experiencing symptoms of balanitis, it's crucial to consult with a healthcare professional for an accurate diagnosis and personalized treatment recommendations.

Risk Factors for Balanitis

Several risk factors can increase the likelihood of developing balanitis. Recognizing these risk factors is essential for understanding the potential causes and taking preventive measures to reduce the risk of balanitis. Here are some common risk factors associated with balanitis:

1. Poor Hygiene

Inadequate Cleaning: Infrequent or improper cleaning of the penis, especially under the foreskin, can lead to the accumulation of smegma (a mixture of oil and dead skin cells) and bacteria, increasing the risk of inflammation and infection.

2. Infections

Bacterial Infections: Exposure to bacteria like Streptococcus or Staphylococcus species due to poor hygiene, minor injuries, or sexual activity can contribute to the development of balanitis.

Yeast Infections (Candidal Balanitis): Factors such as warm and moist environments, use of antibiotics, diabetes, or weakened immune system can promote the overgrowth of Candida species, leading to yeast infections and inflammation.

3. Skin Conditions

Dermatitis: Exposure to irritants (e.g., soaps, detergents, condoms, topical medications) or allergens (e.g., latex, spermicides, personal care products) can cause contact dermatitis or allergic reactions.

Psoriasis or Lichen Planus: Individuals with psoriasis or lichen planus are at higher risk of developing balanitis due to chronic skin inflammation and increased sensitivity to irritants.

4. Irritants

Chemical Irritants: Exposure to chemical irritants from personal care products, medications, or environmental factors can lead to irritation, inflammation, and skin reactions.

Physical Irritants: Friction from tight clothing, condoms, or vigorous sexual activity can cause irritation, discomfort, and increased susceptibility to balanitis.

5. Underlying Health Conditions

Diabetes: Poorly controlled diabetes can impair immune function, elevate glucose levels in the urine, and promote bacterial or fungal growth, increasing the risk of balanitis.

Phimosis: Tight foreskin that cannot be retracted can lead to poor hygiene, trapping of smegma, and increased susceptibility to inflammation and infection.

Sexually Transmitted Infections (STIs): Unprotected sexual activity with an infected partner can increase the risk of contracting STIs that may cause balanitis.

6. Age and Lifestyle Factors

Age: Older men, especially those who are uncircumcised, may be at higher risk due to reduced immune response, decreased elasticity of the foreskin, and increased susceptibility to skin conditions.

Lifestyle Choices: Practices such as smoking, excessive alcohol consumption, or use of recreational drugs can weaken the immune system, impair skin integrity, and contribute to the development of balanitis.

Understanding the risk factors associated with balanitis can help individuals identify potential triggers, take preventive actions, and seek timely medical advice for early diagnosis and treatment. Maintaining good hygiene, practicing safe sex, managing underlying health conditions, avoiding irritants, and adopting a healthy lifestyle are key strategies to reduce the risk of balanitis and promote genital health and well-being. If you or someone you know is experiencing symptoms or risk factors for balanitis, it's essential to consult with a healthcare professional for personalized advice, evaluation, and appropriate management.

Clinical Presentation of Balanitis

The clinical presentation of balanitis can vary depending on the underlying cause, severity, and duration of the inflammation. Common symptoms associated with balanitis include:

Symptoms of Balanitis:

Redness (Erythema)

The affected area, including the foreskin and glans, may appear red or inflamed.

Swelling (Edema)

Swelling of the foreskin and glans can occur, leading to tightness, discomfort, and difficulty retracting the foreskin (phimosis).

Itching (Pruritus)

Persistent itching or irritation of the foreskin and glans can be a common symptom, leading to scratching and further skin damage.

Burning Sensation

A burning or stinging sensation during urination or sexual activity may be present due to inflammation and irritation of the affected area.

Pain or Discomfort

Painful sensations, soreness, or discomfort in the genital area, especially during erection, foreskin retraction, or sexual intercourse.

Discharge

Whitish or yellowish discharge from the penis, particularly in bacterial or fungal infections, may be present.

Odor

Foul-smelling odor from the affected area due to bacterial or fungal overgrowth, especially in cases of poor hygiene or secondary infections.

Ulceration or Sores

Presence of ulcers, blisters, or sores on the foreskin or glans, particularly in cases of severe inflammation, bacterial or viral infections, or underlying skin conditions.

Difficulty Urinating

Pain or discomfort during urination, frequent urination, or other urinary symptoms may occur due to inflammation and irritation of the urethra.

Additional Symptoms:

Systemic Symptoms: In severe or systemic infections, individuals may experience fever, chills, fatigue, or malaise.

Secondary Infections: Complications such as cellulitis (skin infection), abscess formation, or systemic infections may develop if balanitis is left untreated or poorly managed.

Clinical Presentation Based on Types:

Candidal Balanitis: In addition to the above symptoms, individuals with yeast infections may experience a thick, white, cottage cheese-like discharge and increased redness and irritation.

Bacterial Balanitis: Bacterial infections may present with pus-filled lesions, foul-smelling discharge, and worsening inflammation.

Contact Dermatitis: Individuals may have a history of exposure to irritants or allergens, and the symptoms may be localized to the contact area with a distinct pattern of inflammation or rash.

Chronic Balanitis: Symptoms may be recurrent, lasting for an extended period, with periods of exacerbation and remission, and may be associated with underlying conditions like diabetes, psoriasis, or lichen planus.

The clinical presentation of balanitis can vary from mild to severe, with symptoms ranging from localized inflammation and discomfort to systemic complications. Prompt recognition of symptoms, early diagnosis, and appropriate treatment are essential to alleviate symptoms, prevent complications, and promote healing. If you or someone you know is experiencing symptoms suggestive of balanitis, it's crucial to consult with a healthcare professional for an accurate diagnosis and personalized treatment recommendations.

Evaluation and Diagnosis of Balanitis

The evaluation and diagnosis of balanitis involve a comprehensive assessment of the symptoms, medical history, physical examination, and may require additional diagnostic tests to identify the underlying cause and guide appropriate treatment. A healthcare professional, such as a primary care physician, urologist, or dermatologist, typically conducts the evaluation and diagnosis of balanitis.

Evaluation and Diagnostic Steps for Balanitis:

Medical History Assessment

Symptom Review: Detailed questioning about the onset, duration, severity, and progression of symptoms, including redness, swelling, itching, pain, discharge, and urinary symptoms.

Risk Factor Assessment: Inquiry about potential risk factors, such as poor hygiene, recent sexual activity, underlying health conditions (e.g., diabetes), medications, or exposure to irritants or allergens.

Physical Examination

Genital Examination: Visual inspection of the penis, foreskin, and glans for signs of inflammation, redness, swelling, discharge, ulcers, or skin lesions.

Foreskin Retraction: Assessment of foreskin mobility and retractability to evaluate for phimosis or other anatomical abnormalities.

Inguinal Lymph Nodes: Palpation of the inguinal (groin) lymph nodes for swelling, tenderness, or signs of infection.

Microscopic Examination: Collection and microscopic examination of penile swabs or smears to identify bacterial, fungal, or yeast infections.

Culture and Sensitivity Testing: Culture of the penile swab to isolate and identify specific microorganisms responsible for the infection and determine their sensitivity to antibiotics or antifungal agents.

Urinalysis: Urine test to rule out urinary tract infections or other urinary abnormalities associated with balanitis symptoms.

Skin Biopsy (if indicated)

Biopsy: In cases of chronic or recurrent balanitis, skin biopsy may be performed to rule out underlying skin conditions like psoriasis, lichen planus, or malignancies.

Additional Diagnostic Tests (if indicated)

Blood Tests: Blood tests may be conducted to evaluate for systemic conditions like diabetes, HIV, or other underlying health conditions that may contribute to balanitis.

Sexually Transmitted Infection (STI) Testing: Testing for STIs, such as syphilis, herpes, chlamydia, or gonorrhea, if indicated based on the medical history, physical examination, or clinical suspicion.

The evaluation and diagnosis of balanitis require a systematic approach involving a thorough medical history assessment, physical examination, and appropriate diagnostic tests to identify the underlying cause and guide targeted treatment. Early diagnosis and appropriate management are essential to alleviate symptoms, prevent complications, and promote healing. If you or someone you know is experiencing symptoms suggestive of balanitis, it's crucial to consult with a healthcare professional for an accurate diagnosis and personalized treatment recommendations tailored to individual needs and circumstances.

CHAPTER THREE

Treatment Approaches for Balanitis

The treatment of balanitis depends on the underlying cause, severity of symptoms, and individual patient factors. A comprehensive approach involving lifestyle modifications, topical treatments, medications, and, in some cases, surgical interventions may be recommended to manage balanitis effectively. Here are some common treatment approaches for balanitis:

1. Hygiene and Self-Care

Good Hygiene Practices: Maintain proper genital hygiene by cleaning the penis regularly, especially under the foreskin, using mild soap and warm water, and drying the area thoroughly after washing.

Avoid Irritants: Avoid using harsh soaps, perfumed products, or irritating substances that can exacerbate inflammation and irritation of the foreskin and glans.

2. Topical Treatments

Antifungal Creams: Over-the-counter or prescription antifungal creams, such as clotrimazole, miconazole, or ketoconazole, may be used to treat yeast infections (candidal balanitis).

Topical Steroids: Prescription corticosteroid creams or ointments may be prescribed to reduce inflammation, itching, and discomfort associated with allergic or inflammatory balanitis.

Antibacterial Ointments: Topical antibiotics like mupirocin or bacitracin may be used to treat bacterial infections, especially if secondary bacterial infection is present.

3. Oral Medications

Antifungal Medications: Oral antifungal agents, such as fluconazole or itraconazole, may be prescribed for severe or recurrent yeast infections that do not respond to topical treatments.

Antibiotics: Oral antibiotics, such as penicillin, erythromycin, or ciprofloxacin, may be prescribed for bacterial infections or secondary bacterial complications.

Antihistamines: Oral antihistamines, such as cetirizine or loratadine, may be recommended to relieve itching and allergic reactions associated with contact dermatitis.

4. Surgical Interventions

Circumcision: In cases of recurrent balanitis or phimosis (tight foreskin), circumcision may be recommended to reduce the risk of inflammation, improve hygiene, and alleviate symptoms.

Frenuloplasty: Surgical procedure to release or lengthen the frenulum (the band of tissue connecting the foreskin to the glans) to improve foreskin mobility and reduce irritation.

5. Lifestyle and Dietary Modifications

Healthy Diet: Adopting a balanced diet rich in fruits, vegetables, whole grains, lean proteins, and healthy fats can support immune function and overall health.

Blood Sugar Control: Individuals with diabetes should monitor and control blood sugar levels to reduce the risk of recurrent infections and complications.

6. Avoiding Sexual Activity

Temporary Abstinence: Avoiding sexual activity until symptoms resolve completely can prevent further irritation, transmission of infections, and potential complications.

Safe Sex Practices: If sexually transmitted infections (STIs) are suspected or diagnosed, practicing safe sex, using condoms, and informing sexual partners are essential to prevent transmission and re-infection.

The treatment of balanitis is tailored to individual needs, focusing on alleviating symptoms, resolving the underlying cause, and preventing recurrence. Early diagnosis, appropriate management, and adherence to treatment recommendations are essential for successful outcomes. If you or someone you know is experiencing symptoms of balanitis, it's crucial to consult with a healthcare professional for an accurate diagnosis and personalized treatment plan tailored to your specific condition and circumstances.

Prevention Strategies for Balanitis

Prevention strategies for balanitis focus on maintaining good genital hygiene, reducing exposure to irritants and allergens, managing underlying health conditions, and adopting healthy lifestyle habits to minimize the risk of inflammation, infections, and recurrent episodes. Here are some key prevention strategies for balanitis:

1. Good Genital Hygiene

Regular Cleaning: Clean the penis regularly, including the foreskin, using mild soap and warm water. Gently retract the foreskin and rinse thoroughly to remove smegma, bacteria, and other debris.

Proper Drying: Ensure the genital area is dried thoroughly after washing to prevent moisture buildup, which can promote bacterial or fungal growth.

Hygiene After Intercourse: Clean the genital area after sexual activity to remove any potential irritants, lubricants, or semen.

2. Avoid Irritants and Allergens

Gentle Products: Use mild, hypoallergenic soaps, detergents, and personal care products to reduce the risk of skin irritation and allergic reactions.

Avoid Harsh Chemicals: Limit exposure to irritants such as perfumed products, dyes, harsh soaps, or chemicals that can irritate the genital skin.

3. Safe Sexual Practices

Use Condoms: Practice safe sex by using condoms to reduce the risk of sexually transmitted infections (STIs) that can cause balanitis.

Limit Number of Partners: Limit the number of sexual partners and communicate openly about sexual history and STIs to reduce the risk of exposure to infections.

4. Manage Underlying Health Conditions

Control Diabetes: Maintain optimal blood sugar levels through proper diet, exercise, and medication management if you have diabetes, as uncontrolled diabetes can increase the risk of infections and balanitis.

Treat Skin Conditions: Manage underlying skin conditions like psoriasis, eczema, or lichen planus with appropriate treatments and regular follow-up with a dermatologist to prevent flare-ups and complications.

5. Wear Loose-Fitting Clothing

Breathable Fabrics: Choose breathable, natural fabrics like cotton underwear to allow proper airflow and reduce moisture and friction, which can contribute to balanitis.

6. Regular Medical Check-ups

Routine Examinations: Schedule regular medical check-ups with a healthcare professional to monitor genital health, screen for underlying conditions, and identify early signs of balanitis or other genital issues.

7. Healthy Lifestyle Habits

Balanced Diet: Adopt a balanced diet rich in fruits, vegetables, whole grains, lean proteins, and healthy fats to support immune function and overall health.

Regular Exercise: Engage in regular physical activity to maintain a healthy weight, improve circulation, and enhance overall well-being.

Implementing these prevention strategies can help reduce the risk of developing balanitis and promote optimal genital health. By maintaining good hygiene practices, avoiding irritants, practicing safe sex, managing underlying health conditions, and adopting a healthy lifestyle, individuals can minimize the risk of inflammation, infections, and recurrent episodes of balanitis. If you have specific concerns or risk factors for balanitis, it's essential to consult with a healthcare professional for personalized advice, assessment, and recommendations tailored to your individual needs and circumstances.

Complications and Long-Term Effects

Balanitis, if left untreated or poorly managed, can lead to various complications and long-term effects that can impact genital health, quality of life, and overall well-being. Early diagnosis, appropriate treatment, and preventive measures are crucial to minimizing these potential complications. Here are some common complications and long-term effects associated with balanitis:

Complications of Balanitis:

Recurrent Infections

Chronic Balanitis: Persistent or recurrent episodes of balanitis can lead to chronic inflammation and discomfort, requiring prolonged treatment and management.

Secondary Infections: Untreated or inadequately treated balanitis can progress to secondary bacterial, fungal, or viral infections, increasing the severity and duration of symptoms.

Foreskin Problems

Phimosis: Chronic inflammation and scarring from balanitis can lead to tightening of the foreskin (phimosis), making it difficult to retract the foreskin and maintain proper hygiene.

Paraphimosis: Inflammation and swelling of the foreskin can cause the foreskin to become trapped behind the glans, leading to pain, swelling, and potential circulation problems requiring medical intervention.

Penile Scarring and Adhesions

Fibrosis and Scarring: Severe or chronic inflammation can result in fibrosis (scarring) of the foreskin or glans, leading to deformity, discomfort, and functional impairment.

Preputial Adhesions: Inflammation and healing processes can cause the inner layer of the foreskin to adhere to the glans, restricting foreskin mobility and increasing the risk of recurrent balanitis.

Urinary Complications

Urethritis: Inflammation and irritation of the urethra (urethritis) can occur, leading to painful urination, urinary frequency, urgency, or other urinary symptoms.

Sexual Health Concerns

Dyspareunia: Painful intercourse (dyspareunia) can develop due to inflammation, scarring, or discomfort associated with balanitis or related complications.

Sexual Dysfunction: Long-term genital issues, discomfort, or cosmetic changes can impact sexual function, desire, and satisfaction.

Stress and Anxiety: Persistent or recurrent balanitis can cause stress, anxiety, embarrassment, and reduced self-esteem, affecting mental well-being and interpersonal relationships.

Sexual Health Concerns: Fear of transmitting infections, discomfort, or sexual dissatisfaction can lead to sexual avoidance, relationship strain, and emotional distress.

Long-Term Effects:

Chronic Genital Discomfort

Persistent Symptoms: Chronic pain, itching, burning, or discomfort in the genital area can persist, affecting daily activities, sleep, and quality of life.

Reduced Quality of Life

Physical Limitations: Mobility issues, hygiene challenges, and sexual discomfort can limit daily activities, independence, and overall well-being.

Psychosocial Impact: Social withdrawal, relationship difficulties, and emotional distress can occur due to chronic symptoms, cosmetic changes, or sexual health concerns associated with balanitis and its complications.

Understanding the potential complications and long-term effects of balanitis underscores the importance of early diagnosis, appropriate treatment, and preventive strategies to minimize risks, alleviate symptoms, and improve overall genital health and well-being. If you or someone you know is experiencing symptoms or complications related to balanitis, it's crucial to consult with a healthcare professional for accurate diagnosis, tailored treatment, and ongoing management to address individual needs and promote optimal recovery and quality of life.

Conclusion

In conclusion, balanitis is a common inflammatory condition affecting the foreskin and glans of the penis, characterized by redness, swelling, itching, and discomfort. Understanding the causes, risk factors, clinical presentation, and potential complications of balanitis is essential for early diagnosis, appropriate treatment, and preventive measures to maintain genital health and overall well-being.

Effective management of balanitis involves a multifaceted approach, including good genital hygiene, avoidance of irritants and allergens, safe sexual practices, management of underlying health conditions, and lifestyle modifications. Early intervention, accurate diagnosis, and tailored treatment strategies can help alleviate symptoms, prevent complications, and promote healing, enhancing quality of life and sexual health.

Regular medical check-ups, open communication with healthcare providers, and adherence to treatment recommendations are vital for monitoring genital health, addressing concerns, and preventing recurrent episodes or long-term complications associated with balanitis.

If you or someone you know is experiencing symptoms of balanitis or has concerns about genital health, it's essential to consult with a healthcare professional for a comprehensive evaluation, accurate diagnosis, personalized treatment plan, and ongoing support to address individual needs and promote optimal genital health and well-being.

Remember, prioritizing genital hygiene, maintaining a healthy lifestyle, practicing safe sex, and seeking timely medical advice are key to preventing balanitis and maintaining a healthy, active, and fulfilling life. Your genital health matters, and proactive care and attention can make a significant difference in preventing balanitis and related complications, ensuring a safe, satisfying, and confident life journey.

THE END